G. Calvosa

G. Dubois

Rehabilitation in the dynamic stabilization of the lumbosacral spine

G. Calvosa

G. Dubois

Rehabilitation in the dynamic stabilization of the lumbosacral spine

With the contribution: M. Tenucci, C. Giovannini

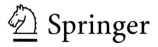 Springer

M.D. Giuseppe Calvosa, spinal surgeon,
Orthopaedic Clinic University of Pisa, Italy

M.D. Gilles Dubois, spinal surgeon,
Neurosurgery of Toulouse, France

M.D. Miria Tenucci, spinal surgeon,
Orthopaedic Clinic University of Pisa, Italy

Dr. Chiara Giovannini
Orthopaedic Clinic University of Pisa, Italy

ISBN 978-3-540-73801-5 Springer Medizin Verlag Heidelberg

Bibliografische Information der Deutschen Bibliothek
The Deutsche Bibliothek lists this publication in Deutsche Nationalbibliographie;
detailed bibliographic data is available in the internet at http://dnb.ddb.de.

Springer Medizin Verlag
springer.com
© Springer Medizin Verlag Heidelberg 2008

The use of general descriptive names, registered names, trademarks, etc. in this publications does not imply, even in the absence of a specific statement, that such names are exempt from the relevant protective laws and regulations and therefore free for general use.

Product liability: The publishers cannot guarantee the accuracy of any information about dosage and application contained in this book. In every individual case the user must check such information by consulting the relevant literature.

SPIN 12097241
Typesetting: TypoStudio Tobias Schaedla, Heidelberg
Printing: Stürtz GmbH, Würzburg

18/5135 – 5 4 3 2 1 0

Preamble

In the past decade, thanks to new and sophisticated instrumental research like the MRI, CT and discography, we have been able to focus better on degenerative pathologies, so that we can now discuss discal bulging, micro-instability (both fragmentary and plurisegmentary), soft stenosis etc.

In addition, the greater development of surgical techniques has allowed us to improve the treatment of these pathologies, of which the one that has aroused most interest in the context of non-fusion is the dynamic stabilization of the lumbar spine. As we all know, in the orthopaedic field, in order to obtain good results, it is necessary to have the proper surgical indications and precise surgical techniques associated with attentive phases of rehabilitation.

I believe, that this publication, which describes the indications and the various phases of technical rehabilitation to be used after surgical treatment of lumbar degenerative spine, represents a work of fundamental importance that is clearly useful to those interested in this area of orthopaedics.

I am certain that this monograph will be widely and justifiably successful.

G. GUIDO
Chief Orthopaedic Clinic University of Pisa

Contents

Introduction

In the musculoskeletal system, the spine has the difficult task of ensuring the stability of the trunk and supporting the upper extremity girdles and pelvic girdle. At times, these functions are altered and compromised as a result of degenerative, traumatic, neoplastic and other pathologies.

The efficiency and equilibrium in the distribution of work loads, in both antigravity statics and mobility, are determined by the co-ordination of the various segments comprising the spine, i.e. the functional units.

The term spinal functional unit refers to the complex of two adjacent vertebrae and the interposed intervertebral disc. The functional units are stacked between them and comprise the spinal articular complex.

Until recently in the field of vertebral surgery, many diseases were managed with surgery of instrumented vertebral stabilization and bone fusion (arthrodesis). Fusion always offered valid and safe results, although at the expense of the abolition of the motility of the spine section which was being operated upon. A review of the surgical cases after 5-10 years demonstrated an overloading of the areas adjoining the arthrodesis area with formation of herniated discs, bone sclerosis and ever-present pain and soreness.

For this reason, when treating degenerative diseases of the lumbosacral spine, the Orthopaedic Clinic of the S. Chiara Hospital in Pisa introduced the Dynesys lumbosacral spine dynamic neutralization system to treat patients and spinal diseases with selected indications.

This is a non-fusion flexible system with transpedicular screws and an flexible connector for dynamic stabilization; it is a new method for treating the degenerative disease of the lumbosacral spine which has been developed in the past few years and preserves motility at the treated levels.

While allowing for movement of the segment at all levels, the Dynesys provides stability to the functional unit, which attains a condition of physiological function compared with the rigid stabilization-arthrodesis.

This publication presents a rehabilitation protocol with physical therapy which we adapted to patients who underwent this surgery.

The protocol used in patients who had dynamic stabilization surgery at the Orthopaedic Clinic of the S. Chiara Hospital in Pisa boasted rapid recovery times and brilliant results. This study was conducted on 30 cases: 10 men and 20 women, mean age 42 years, evaluated using the VAS scale and the Oswestry Low Back Pain Disability Questionnaire, with follow-up of 1 to 4 years after surgery.

The pathologies treated are: disc bulging and micro-instability with lumbar pain and irritating sciatica; herniated disc and micro-instability of one level with irritating lumbar-sciatic pain; spondy-losis with stenosis affecting at least two levels; degenerative spondylolisthesis of one level up to grade 2; repeated surgery on a herniated disc at one or two levels; rotational scoliosis of moderate grade in adults.

Concepts of Biomechanics

2.1 Biomechanics of the lumbar spine

The lumbar spine, located between the chest area and the pelvis, needs to meet two apparently inconsistent static and dynamic requirements: from a static standpoint, resistance to loads and transmission of forces; from a dynamic standpoint, movement. The lumbar area is thus an element of transmission and adaptation, like an elastic shock absorber, which feels the impact of any overlying or underlying disequilibrium.

The role of the intervertebral disc, cornerstone of spinal statics, is to absorb shocks and transmit the load through the vertebral bodies as well as to allow movement of the adjacent functional units. It is composed of three parts: a nucleus pulposus, a highly hydrated central gelatinous mass, the fibrous ring, a circular fibrous part which surrounds and contains the nucleus pulposus, and the superficial portion of the vertebral plate, made of a cartilaginous layer which covers the upper and lower surfaces of the intervertebral disc [6].

When the disc is subject to a vertical compression force, it demonstrates an adequate amount of resistance to the application of small loads and a greater resistance to greater loads which, however, decrease immediately after the first break. The paravertebral muscles contract and increase tone, even in the ring. The pressure increases in the nucleus pulposus and also extends to the fibrous ring, the most internal fibres of which tighten and in turn resist the applied force, and superficial portion of the vertebral plates.

The compression forces on the disc cause a radial bulging of the disc itself which is more prominent in the compression area.

Together with the position of the spine in space, the lumbar lordosis affects the amount of intradiscal pressure, which is higher when sitting (particularly with the flexed trunk) than when standing, as shown by the Nachenson studies [14, 19].

Intra-abdominal pressure (IAP) also plays an important role in spinal statics.

The layout of the lumbar spine also affects weight distribution between the anterior and posterior portions of the spine: greater anterior load with reduced lordosis, greater posterior compression with increased lordosis.

Statically, the presence of curves in the spine increases the resistance of the spine to axial compression stress. Lumbar lordosis is thus essential to reduce the load on the intervertebral discs. The physiological lordosis is also maintained due to the shape of the lumbar discs, which are higher in the anterior than in the posterior portion. Because of the lordosis, the intervertebral discs are subjected to greater pressure, which tends to maintain the nucleus gel in a more anterior position and to prevent its posterior protrusion. The maintenance of the lumbar curvature, intra-abdominal pressure and tone of the paravertebral muscles actually strengthen the spine, and are essential to protect the spine when lifting weights. On the contrary, a reduced lordosis promotes stress against the intervertebral discs. Dynamically, mathematical studies find in the physiological lordosis the element required to achieve proper anterior flexion since only then are the intrinsic musculature, posterior ligaments and the intervertebral joints put in tension for the purposes of the movement arc. Lumbar lordosis is thus an important element in both static and dynamic physiology. An increase, a reduction or altered distribution of this spinal curve inevitably changes the functionality of the spine and can promote the occurrence of subsequent mechanical stress, mostly at the disc level. In conclusion, we believe that during the pursuit of vertebral surgery it is extremely important to maintain, whenever possible, the reconstruction and the sagittal balance [12].

Vertebral Degeneration

3.1 Pathogenesis of disc degeneration

The structure of the intervertebral disc generally remains unchanged until the second decade of life. Regressive changes subsequently occur with age. These morphological and biochemical alterations are more frequent and prominent in the lower lumbar segments, which are subject to the highest pressure stress due to the motion of the lumbosacral hinge.

Body weight, lumbar lordosis, functional overloads, demanding work on the spine, abnormalities in the differentiation of the lumbosacral passage, connective tissue diseases which predispose to degenerative diseases, idiopathic instabilities and early senescence phenomena can, even at an early age, cause disc degenerations which generally accompany the aging process. A gross examination demonstrates loss of the mucoid aspect of the nucleus which becomes dry, solid, even friable, with fibrocartilaginous characteristics. This is followed by the conversion of the fibrous ring into a rigid, fibrous, non-elastic structure which tends to become the seat of fissures and lacerations. These fissures result from small degenerative foci of the fibrillar structure which progressively converge towards one another, becoming increasingly wider. Furthermore, they are distributed over the entire fibrous ring with a certain predominance in the posterior area. Histological examination evidences a progressive reduction in the number of cells; it also highlights the thickening and crystallization of collagen fibres. The basic substance composed of mucopolysaccharides tends to diminish progressively while losing consistency in the interfibrillar distribution, which causes tissue dehydration and thus a defective nutrition of the disc due to defective metabolic exchanges with accumulation of waste and lipids. The resulting loss of the elastic properties of the disc in its two components (nucleus pulposus and fibrous ring) is responsible for the mechanical damage (◻ Fig. 3.1).

The regressive changes in molecular structures are accompanied by changes in the architectonic structures of the disc tissue. The ring's laminae, adjacent to the pulpy nucleus, change their medial concavity into convexity as a result of the fibrocartilaginous retraction of the nucleus, while external convexity is increased in peripheral laminae, thus causing a posterior protrusion, called bulging. Finally, the interposed laminae will be oriented parallel to the major axis. The involutional adaptation of the disc prevents the nucleus pulposus from sending impulses to the fibrous ring, thus cancelling the primary characteristic of the intervertebral discs, i.e. amortizing and redistributing the loads received, allowing the mechanical forces to act directly on the fibrocartilage and damage it, and promoting the irritating bone neoproduction of the vertebral plates (osteophytes and spur tractions) [4, 17] (◻ Fig. 3.2).

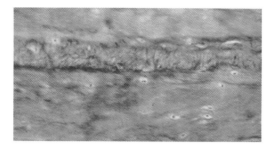

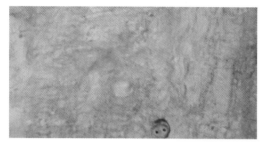

◘ Fig. 3.1. a Healthy intervertebral disc. **b** Degenerated intervertebral disc

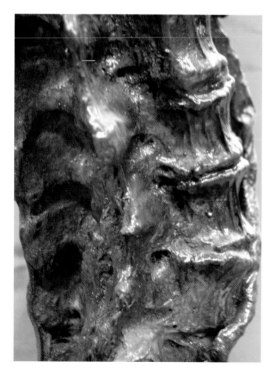

◘ Fig. 3.2. Anatomical preparation showing an advanced disc degeneration with plate bone sclerosis

3.2   Vertebral instability

It is not yet fully clear whether disc degeneration leads to vertebral instability or whether the latter leads to disc degeneration. Biomechanic studies carried out by Panjabi in 1982 demonstrated that rachis is extremely elastic when it is subjected to small compressive forces and increases its rigidity as the weight-bearing increases.

This concept can be expressed (◘ Fig. 3.3) by a graph that takes into consideration two parameters: the range of movement (ROM) and the neutral zone (NZ) where the NZ is the portion of ROM where the rachis has the minimal resistency to movement, i.e that zone where the rachis is mostly elastic [21, 27].

All the elements of FSU (functional spinal unit) (disc, articular, ligaments) contributed to the stability of the system and the mutation of every one of these elements, whether for traumatic or degenerative causes, upsets the delicate equilibrium the stability and physiological rigidity of FSU.

In order to make a simple comparison, the weight-bearing movement graph (◘ Fig 3.3) can be considered as similar to the movement made by a ball in a glass.

Inside the NZ the ball moves easily, but requires a major effort to move outside when the edges are higher; so the smaller the NZ, the more stable the column.

When one of the elements of the FSU is altered, the NZ increases and the ball moves easily beyond the pain-free movement zone (◘ Fig 3.4).

In those cases where the rachis has lost its physiological rigidity, and even phyisiological load-bearing movements determine pain, we can speak of instability.

Dynamic stabilization permits us to neutralize one or more adjacent FSU. The use of transpedicular conic screws and of a pretensioned elastic spacer permits us to stabilize the damaged functional unit, thus re-establishing the range of controlled movement; thanks to neutralization, it can also absorb non-physiological loads, in both compression and flex extension.

Lumbar vertebral instability is a degenerative or microtraumatic disease, characterized by postural pain that is dependent upon the body position, which occurs at certain times of the day; for example, after a long standing position or after having sat for a lengthy period of time in front of a computer. It is occasionally accompanied (this is observed mostly in the forms associated with a stenosis of the vertebral or foraminal canal) by torpor or a sense of sleepiness and weakness in the lower extremities.

Degenerative instability generally affects the last lumbar vertebrae from L4 to S1. The wear and ageing of the intervertebral disc and osteoligamentous portions cause a loss of articular solidity, reducing the space for the nervous structures, specifically the medullary cone and lumbosacral nerve roots. Subject to a considerable stress, the nerve

roots respond with pain and occasionally with motor limitations. Stenosis of the intervertebral foramen can occur due to congenital shortness of the peduncles, intraforaminal bulging or phenomena of intervertebral arthrosis. All these abnormal conditions lead to pathological states which can occur individually or combined together.

Osteoporosis can aggravate this clinical picture, with the potential addition of a vertebral crushing.

The morphological changes sustained by the osteoligamentous structures cause a reduction in the volume of the vertebral canal, with disc protrusion, a reduction in the lateral recess and the conjugate foramens, and with pain and deficit for the medulla and/or nerve roots.

It is possible to identify and divide the development of a degenerative spondylosis (Kirkaldy Wyllis) into three stages, resulting from the intervertebral instability which leads to the anatomical-pathological states of the acquired stenosis.

The first stage is characterized by the degeneration of the intervertebral disc and radicular irritation.

The second stage is characterized by loss of height, development of an intervertebral instability with lumbar pain and an occasional irritating radicular disease or a lack of force and reflexes.

One then reaches the final stage of acquired stenosis which implicates a clinical status involving continuous or intermittent radicular syndrome and motor deficits at one or more levels with the classic medullary claudicatio intermittens [13].

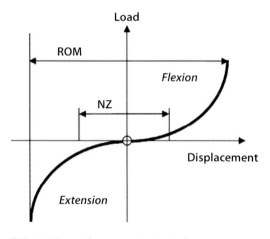

☐ **Fig. 3.3.** Range of movement and neutral zone

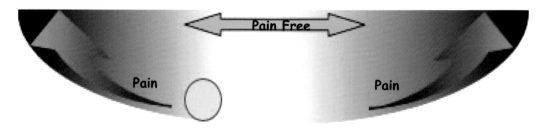

☐ **Fig. 3.4.** Simple comparison of Fig. 3

Surgical Treatment: From Stabilization-Arthrodesis to Non-Fusion

The conventional stabilization of the lumbosacral spine is based on the now obsolete and consolidated surgical technique of arthrodesis.

This method, devised by the American R.H. Hibbs in 1911, is based essentially on the surgical procedure of cruentation, using gouges, scalpels and rongeurs of the posterior bone surface of the spine so as to induce a repair mechanism for the formation of bone callus with suppression of the movement of one or more functional units [11].

In the 1960s, the posterior arthrodesis technique was significantly improved by Watkins and Wiltse, who extended the decorticated surfaces to include the spinal processes and transverses, giving rise to the posterolateral arthrodesis. The arthrodesis, which is essentially a biological technique, was combined with the use of containing casts to encourage the formation of bone callus. These casts were worn for a variable period of 5-6 months until maturation of the arthrodesis area [26].

An important step forward in the field of vertebral surgery was accomplished with the 1960's design of the American P. Harrington of a universal instrument of sublaminar hooks and stabilizing bars. This system introduced the philosphy of distraction and internal stabilization in spinal surgery and combined it with the biological fusion of arthrodesis (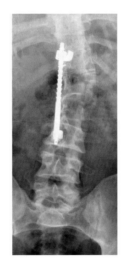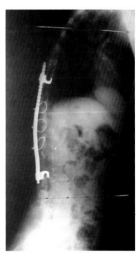Fig. 4.1).

◻ **Fig. 4.1.** Scoliosis treated with Harrington-Luque

Scoliosis surgery took particular advantage of this technique, and expanded it throughout the world, with brilliant results.

There was also a remarkable attempt by the Mexican E.R. Luque to design a multisegment sublaminar fixation method with metal wires, which is still indicated in neurological scoliosis [15].

The most important change in the history of modern vertebral surgery occurred in the 1970s due to Roy Camille, who designed fixation with transpedicular screws, which remains today the keystone of the stabilization systems [22].

Substantial progress in this technique was, however, made by Cotrel and Debousset in France, who suggested that scoliosis, as a curve developed along three planes, requires more complex instruments to correct the curves in three dimensions [5].

Thanks to the use of the transpedicular fixation, it was possible to take the most advantage of the combined technique of stabilization and arthrodesis in most vertebral diseases.

Since the 1980s, together with the expansion of this technique, its limitations have become obvious: the results of the instrumented arthrodesis deteriorated about 7 years after surgery in 42% of the cases.

Clinical and radiographical studies had documented a recurrence of the degenerative phenomenon above and below the arthrodesis area, in the so-called junctional area, due to the use of excessively rigid stabilization (◘ Fig. 4.2).[1, 3, 8, 9].

The need to preserve the movement of the spinal functional unit, avoiding the articular block-age of the arthrodesis and complications in the junctional areas, was first reported by the French colleagues Brondsarde and Graaf, who opened the door to the development of non-fusion techniques.

In the 1980s the concept of dynamic segmental non-harmonies was born, i.e. abnormal spinal hyperlaxity or hypermobility, similar to modern instability, for which the above-mentioned authors proposed ligamentous orthoses with interspinal pads and elastic bands on transpedicular screws.

With regards to vertebral instability, J. Senegas also developed the concept of »ligamentoplasty« in the case of disc dehydration with dysfunction and wear of the interarticulars [23].

These first attempts to offer an elastic stability to the spinal functional unit resulted in a high percentage of failures due to the difficulty in developing suitable indications or due to the incapacity of these first instruments, which were excessively elastic, to assure the rigidity of the functional units.

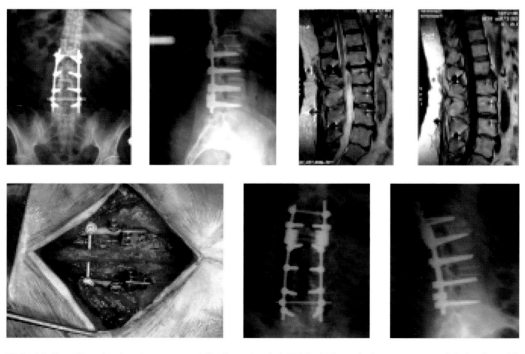

◘ **Fig. 4.2.** Case of junctional syndrome post-stabilization-arthrodesis L2-L5 which required surgery to extend the implant with transpeduncular screws in the L1-L2 junctional area with dominance and new decompression of the canal at L5-S1

New non-fusion instruments have been developed in the past few years:

- interspinous spacers (DIAM of J. Taylor, Wallis of J. Senegas), which will be addressed below (◘ Fig. 4.3) [16].
- Dynesys System, leader of dynamic stabilization, a new technique successfully used since 2001 at the Orthopaedic Clinic of the University of Pisa, which will be addressed in the following section.

The DIAM is a silicone spacer which can be inserted while saving the interspinal ligament so as to operate as a tension band. It maintains the rigidity of the posterior compartment of the functional unit, and therefore it is indicated when the maintaince of the dimension of the radicular canal is desired. If the intent is to go beyond maintaining a static position in the diameter of the radicular canal in order to look for better stability, one must necessarily achieve a kyphotization of the spinal segment with level rigidity and inversion of the physiological lordosis. Therefore one cannot talk of this device, as with all interspinal devices, as a true stabilizer, since it lacks a stabilizing force; therefore it is a spacer.

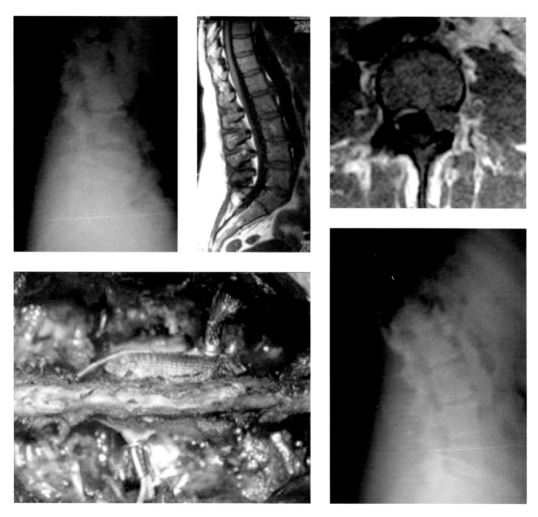

◘ **Fig. 4.3.** Case of massive L4-L5 hernia which required surgical removal of hernia and disc clean-up with subsequent implantation of a DIAM-type interspinal spacer

5

Dynamic Stabilization with the Dynesys System

The vertebral stabilization system (Dynesys) [7, 24, 25], designed in France by Gilles Dubois approximately 15 years ago, and successfully used since 2001 at the Orthopaedic Clinic of the S. Chiara Hospital in Pisa, is composed of transpedicular conical screws, a polycarbonate urethane spacer and a polyethylene tensioning cord (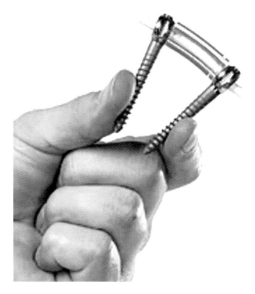 Fig. 5.1). It works as a real shock absorber, so that it not only enlarges the functional unit, re-opening its intervertebral foramen, but, with the pretensioning achieved in the operating field, restores force and stability to the disc, enhancing the biological possibilities of curing the degenerative disease.

Its use results from the need for early intervention on the degenerative cascade to restore physiological rigidity and stability to the spinal functional unit while preserving the natural mobility of the spinal segment before the effects of the degeneration become irreversible. More particularly, it is in stage II of Kirkaldy-Willis, when the height loss is obvious and the patient develops vertebral instability with chronic lumbar pain and pain accross and/or irritating sciatica, that one can successfully operate with dynamic stabilization, the Dynesys System (Fig. 5.2).

With Dynesys, one can put in dynamic neutralization one or more adjacent functional spinal units and, through the transpedicular conical screws, this system succeeds in stabilizing the damaged func-

Fig. 5.1. Dynesys System

tional unit, restoring the range of controlled movements. With neutralization, non-physiological loads can be absorbed in compression and flexion-extension. In this way, the functional segment can be brought back to a physiological situation restoring elasticity to the system, as stated by Panjabi [21,25].

In these cases, the dynamic stabilization (almost always without revising the sac and roots) restores disc height and suppresses the disc-root conflict while maintaining the functional unit's capacity to move (■ Fig. 5.3).

From 2001 to 2004, our cases of micro-instability treated with dynamic stabilization in neutralization without fusion include 30 patients: 10 men and 20 women, mean ages 42 years. All the subjects were evaluated with the VAS scale and the Oswestry Low Back Pain Questionnaire before and after surgery. The follow-up ranged from 1 to 4 years (■ Fig. 5.4).

We encountered ten cases of disc bulging and micro-instability with lumbar pain and irritating sciatica at L4-L5; three cases of herniated disc and micro-instability of one level with irritating lumbago-sciatica at L4-L5; six cases of spondylosis with related stenosis at two levels; three cases of spondylosis with related stenosis and lumbar pain-cruralgia and sciatica at three levels; six cases of

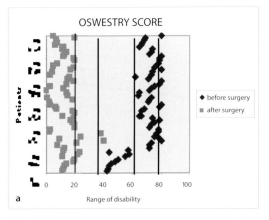

a

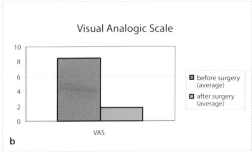

b

■ **Fig. 5.4. a** Oswestry score. **b** Visual analogic scale

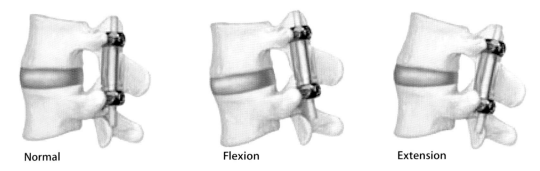

■ **Fig. 5.2.** Dynesys stabilization system attached bilaterally to spine. (Photo courtesy of Zimmer, Inc.)

Normal   Flexion   Extension

■ **Fig. 5.3.** Dynamic neutralization with Dynesys

repeated surgery on a herniated disc at two levels L4-L5 and L5-S1 with micro-instability.

All the cases were studied with MRI after at least 1 year. We obtained 70% rehydratations with over 90% very good and good results.

Reported below are other important cases of our follow-up which allow the assessment of the restoration of disc space and segment stabilization, while preserving the functional unit's capacity to move, and the rehydration of the intervertebral disc, always with remission of the painful symptoms (◘ Fig. 5.5).

The high success percentage, in over 90% of the cases, was certainly due to the thorough pre-operative examination, the study of the case in both its clinical aspect and its imaging and the proper performance of the original operating technique. In dynamic stabilization, remarkable progress in rehabilitation treatment, in addition to surgery, was the routine introduction of the Wiltse surgical approach in cases which do not involve an intermediate time of canal and/or radicular revision.

In the Wiltse posterolateral approach [28], the muscles are preserved. With this method one actually proceeds in a blunt manner into the septum which divides the the muscles of the more medial compartment from those of the more lateral compartment up to the articular transverse, through a transmuscular approach of the sacrospinal muscles (◘ Fig. 5.6).

The patient evidences less bleeding both during and after surgery along with less pain. The patient can thus be mobilized earlier.

Using the Dynesys L.I.S. (Less Invasive Surgery) instrument, we can dynamically stabilize one or more levels and put the patient on his or her feet on the first day, thus starting rehabilitation much earlier than with patients who had rigid stabilization, which always required longer rehabilitation and the passage of months before returning to work and a normal life style (◘ Fig. 5.7).

The non-fusion surgical techniques, supported by efficient instruments and an elegant and simple surgical approach, will always be more accepted among spine surgeons. The possibility of intervening earlier on the disc degeneration, the full respect of the intervertebral disc and articulars, the extraordinary capacity of the disc to rehydrate and the full respect of the functional unit's movement are definitely a step forward in the search for better results with this difficult disease.

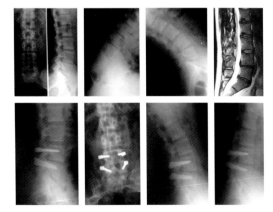

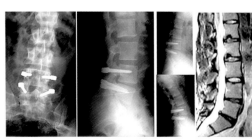

◘ **Fig. 5.5.** 34-year-old man with herniated disc L4-L5 with irritating lumbar pain. The stabilization in neutralization with the removal of the herniated disc is performed

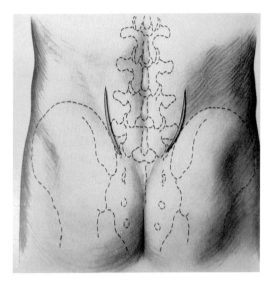

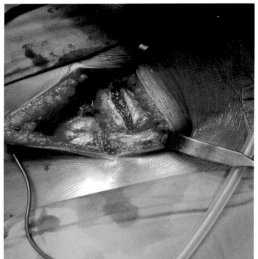

Fig. 5.6. Wiltse posterolateral approach for dynamic stabilizations without incidental time of radicular and/or canal revision

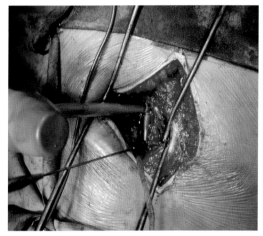

Fig. 5.7. Modified Wiltse surgical approach; Dynesys system; L.I.S. technique, at level L4-L5

6

Rehabilitation in Spinal Stabilization-Arthrodesis

The patient who undergoes »conventional« rigid lumbar stabilization surgery sustains considerable post-traumatic stress due to the wide skeletization with loosening of the paravertebral muscular masses, the arthrodesis with cruentation of the laminae and articular processes, and often also the incidental time for sampling autologous bone and iliac wing or spinous processes from the bed subject to arthrodesis. All these results in very aggresssive and mutilating surgical times which cause permanent structural dysfunction of the spine, the significance of which varies with the number of segments fused (◘ Fig. 6.1).

Therefore rehabilitation should take into account the articular limitations which will remain from the stabilization-arthrodesis and prevent possible postoperative complications, protecting as much as possible the adjacent discs which are knowingly subject to overloading and degeneration.

Surgery with the conventional medial approach, with skeletization of the paravertebral muscles from their compartments (right and left) requires, after surgery, a few days of bed rest. The patient is placed in orthostatic position during the 3rd and 4th days. There should be a long monitoring period of the surgical levels so as to form a significant muscular scar and to achieve (approximately 5 months after surgery) the total loss of the articular motility of the stabilized and arthrodesized segments.

Years after surgery, the electromyography of the paravertebral muscles evidences reduced or absent muscular electric activity due to wide areas of fibrosis.

In the first few days after surgery, when the patient cannot stand, the physical therapist should teach only exercises of mobilization in the lower extremities so as to avoid the complications due to immobilization, such as circulatory problems, sores, etc.

In the initial stages, it is essential to use a soft approach to movement with respect of the patient's pain and to alleviate this, if necessary, with antalgics and physical therapy (massages, TENS, etc.)

In the acute stage, during the first 2 or 3 weeks after surgery, the physical therapist should show the patient the proper way to use the crutches and the correct manner for wearing the fabric and steel corset. Upon discharge, the patient should be given instructions on the movements to avoid and advice on the management of daily household activities.

Proper rehabilitation starts in the stable stage (when the wound is healed and the pain reduced). This takes place in thermal stations or simply in rehabilitation centres and lasts approximately 2 weeks.

During the rehabilitation stage in thermal stations, the patient undergoes sessions of hydrokinesitherapy, in a swimming pool, for 1 hour each day, and kinesitherapy in the gym for 2 hours each day, in 15-day cycles.

At the same centre the patient can take advantage of other physical therapy resources based upon the requirements, which vary from one case to the other. For example, if the scar causes a feeling of tension in segmentary movement, loosening can be achieved with specific massage.

The first therapeutic objective is to improve load distribution. Regardless of the number of segments involved in the vertebral artrodesic fusion, it is useful to strengthen the functions: the lordosis, with the reconstruction of a correct sagittal balance

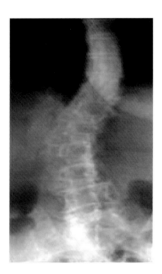
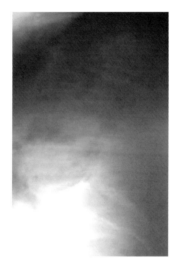
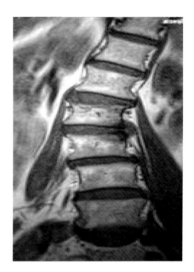
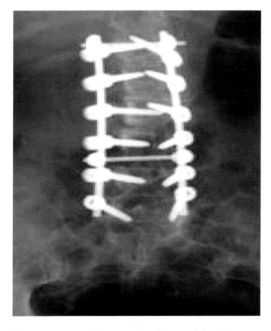
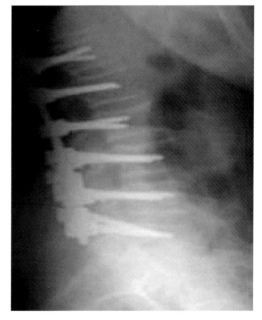

◘ **Fig. 6.1.** Long stabilization-arthrodesis in adult scoliosis

which allows axial resistance to load, to regain, as much as possible, the muscular tone of paravertebral muscles and the hip extension, which will compensate for the spine's reduced mobility.

In the first stage, emphasis is placed on postural treatment in discharge, with exercises in the swimming pool or gym.

The rehabilitation protocol in the swimming pool includes a series of exercises of hydrokinesitherapy, performed in a group for 1 hour each day under the direction of a physical therapist.

Subsequently, to reinforce the static function and to best strengthen the musculature after extensive skeletization and loosenings, exercises of active kinesitherapy are performed in the gym.

Exercises of stabilization with the Swiss ball which allow a proprioceptive approach are of a crucial importance. Exercises of antero-retroversion and lateralization of the pelvis are performed with the ball.

To maintain a wider flexion-extension of the spine, which surgery has reduced by 40-50%, the patient should have access to exercises of segmentary mobilization and soft overall gymnastics. To avoid overloading the discs adjacent to surgery, it is necessary that the segments adjacent to those fused be elastic to accompany the stress during motion. As already stated, the lost extension of the lumbar spine can be compensated by the hip's extension. The lumbar flexion which is no longer possible can be compensated by that of other spinal segments and increased elasticity of the ischio-crurals.

These results are better achieved with proprioceptive exercises, passive articular mobilization, but mostly with stretching.

Rotational movements should be avoided until arthrodesis is fully consolidated, and this, on the average, requires another 6 months after surgery.

Rehabilitation in Dynamic Stabilization with the Dynesys System

The dynamic stabilization with Dynesys, which provides for the introduction of transpedicular screws in lateral position with full respect of the joints, together with the abolition of skeletisation and the total abolition of muscular detachment and consequent preserved mobility of the spine, ensures a faster recovery after surgery.

The patient who undergoes dynamic stabilization with Dynesys through the intermuscular lateral approach, can get up already on the first day following surgery.

The Wiltse blunt intermuscular approach, with the total lack of skeletization moments through the detachment of the paravertebral muscular masses with respect to posterior interarticular joints, capsules and ligaments, and lack of arthrodesization of laminae and processes, allows quick, bloodless stabilization surgery (◘ Fig. 7.1).

The reduced whimpers of the patient after surgery, together with the reduced pain associated with the lumbar spine, result in earlier possible mobilization. Therefore, as early as the first day, although only to the extent allowed for proper healing of the muscles and skin, the patient can comply with the first indications of the physical therapists.

The pain caused by surgery can be alleviated in the first few days with analgetics.

The physical therapist should possess maximum information from the surgeon so as to gain precise knowledge of the type of surgery performed, the potential technical alternatives used, and immediately adapt his or her intervention to the patient's psychological profile. Some patients are more motivated to resume their activities earlier, while others, more insecure because of their fear of having sustained permanent injury and residual postoperative pain, tend not to move the spine.

It is up to the physical therapist to educate the former towards progressive resumption of movement and to not prematurely overload the spine before it has acquired the support of suitable musculature, and to help the second group to regain trust in movement, explaining the benefits inherent in the Dynesys system, making them aware of their own capacity to move the surgical structures without pain or danger. The resumption of normal daily activities should be encouraged immediately and made the least traumatic possible, even for those who live in close contact with the patient.

From the very first days, the patient should be given instructions as to how to sit properly and which auxiliary devices to use, and should also be given information on standing positions and basic ergonomic behaviours.

As early as the first stage of rehabilitation, i.e. in the first 2 weeks following surgery, it is important to promptly start a few perceptive and proprioceptive exercises to »awaken« the lumbar stabilizing function (simple exercises can also be taught after a few days).

The use of the Dynesys system and the intermuscular approach allows for early performance of muscular re-awakening exercises which feature several benefits, including: not finding the back muscles unprepared at the time of the abandonment of the lumbar band and not encouraging the patient to delegate the strength and stabilizing function of his or her back to an auxiliary device. Extended use of the lumbar band could mean making the patient dependent thereon.

The second stage of rehabilitation starts when the patient reaches a condition of stability which allows him or her to resume all physiological movements, without excessive pain or fear. Once the suture stitches are removed and the wound is fully healed, even water rehabilitation is indicated, since it allows for movements under conditions of gravitational no-load.

Therefore it is preferable to choose a centre equipped with both a gym and a swimming pool.

The vertebral function is to ensure simultaneously rigid support of the body, movement and protection of the spinal medulla. The regulation of this function is achieved by the articular and muscular mechanoceptors and nociceptors, afferent and efferent nervous pathways, arthrodynamic and arthrostatic reflexes, regulation and control nervous centres. These systems work automatically and cannot be voluntarily controlled.

A spine affected with degenerative disc disease and subsequently subjected to a traditional stabilization procedure generally displays disorders of the proprioceptive afferences or interference of nociceptive afferences which can change or suspend arthrokinetic reflexes and motor systems for long periods. The use of the technique described above allows the restoration of a physiological condition and avoids the permanent alteration or dysfunction of movement which remains after arthrodesis.

The general objectives of the rehabilitation of the patient with dynamic stabilization are: improvement in load distribution, restoration of proper static-dynamic automatisms, strengthening of the static function and improvement of load resistance.

Proprioceptive exercises, such as oscillating ball or tables, and exercises in the swimming pool are useful in reaching these goals.

The practice of hydrokinesitherapy [2] at the beginning of treatment causes the patient to feel better even on the ground. He or she can actually use the ease and difficulty which he or she finds in water exercise to obtain the easiest and safest motor conditions on the ground, thereby achieving autonomy more rapidly and consequently acquiring further motivation to continue treatment. One thus mobilizes the body segment affected by surgery in a way which is made easier by immersion in hot water, with the advantage that hot water helps to alleviate pain, reduces muscular spasm and increases tissue elasticity.

Group exercises in the swimming pool offer a socializing role in addition to a specific physical function. They are actually simple exercises performed together so as to put the patient at ease and to encourage the beginning of the exercise program for the spine.

Unfortunately, it is not always possible for the patient to follow the rehabilitation sessions in the swimming pool for various reasons, whether they be physical (incontinence, menstruation, or disease, all contra-indications) or psychological (fear, shame etc.). In these cases, the work in the gym becomes more important and can be supplemented with the help of the therapy master, »the third hand of the therapist«, the link between passive and active exercises.

In the gym, the sessions are more customized, and the relationship between the therapist and the patient is intensified. In fact, the physical therapist adapts the rehabilitation plan to the requirements and capacity of each individual patient, selecting the most suitable exercises.

At this stage, it is valuable to use the Overall Postural Rehabilitation, which eliminates painful symptoms while achieving a real reprogramming of the automatic function of the spine's muscles.

While the therapist teaches the patient how to perform the exercises, he should simulate them. Furthermore, the exercises proposed should be primarily symmetrical for the purpose of recreating a proper functional equilibrium of the general movement of the spine.

The physical therapist should keep in mind the objective of the gym work, which is not just muscular strengthening, but also strengthening of the muscular function. This actually includes the proper static-dynamic co-ordination, posture maintenance, capacity to reach maximum spine extension, excentric control of motion and response to unexpected stress. Therefore, it is not necessary to perform analytical strengthening, but one should look for the re-equilibrium of all the forces acting on the spine, thus achieving true neuromotor reprogramming.

For this purpose, the work program should include proprioceptive exercises for the purpose of facilitating the subject's perception and for retraining lumbar stabilization in the passage between opposite movements, within the neutral zone.

At the end of each session at the gym, stretching exercises for the recovery of muscular flexibility are very useful. In fact, the superficial layers of the psoas, the ischio-crurals, and the medial and superficial layers of the posterior spinal musculature are predisposed by their natural function to hypertonia and rigidity.

Finally, it is advisable that the patient undergoes, at this stage, regular massage sessions. These will avoid the muscular contractures due to the intense physical activity for which the muscles are not prepared and to prepare the musculature itself to perform the requested work.

One should not neglect the psychological effects of those techniques which help the patient to remain calm and to trust vis-a-vis the physical therapist, thus relaxing in a difficult situation. If the scar causes a feeling of tension or tends to create adherence to the underlying tissues, loosening massages can be helpful.

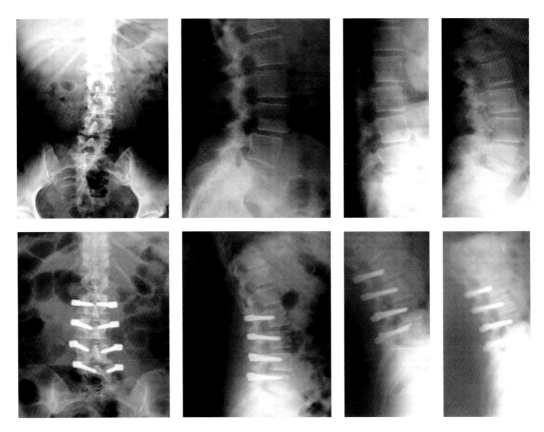

◘ **Fig. 7.1.** Patient with mild degenerative scoliosis and instability treated with Dynesys at three levels

7.1 First Stage of Rehabilitation

In the first, acute, stage, which lasts approximately 2 weeks, it is advisable for the patient to wear fabric and steels corsets and to use auxiliary devices such as a walker to begin mobilization again, either in the hospital under the guidance of the physical therapist or at home, upon discharge.

The physical therapist guides the patient in walking exercises on flat surfaces and on stairs, teaching the patient how to use crutches properly and giving him or her instructions on the movements to avoid in the first few days.

At this stage, the main therapeutic objective is to restore the proper static-dynamic automatisms of the spine, with the fundamental purpose of recovering the load-bearing capacity and motoricity.

One should not neglect to progressively reduce the time of use of the lumbar band, mostly during performance of the most protected daily activities and as the stabilization exercises progress, maintaining it during performance of the most stressful and risky activities.

The exercises to »re-activate« abdominal musculature are:

– **Diaphragmatic Respiration.** The patient is instructed to put one hand on his or her chest and one on the abdomen to make sure that the chest remains immobile during breathing and that only the abdomen moves.
– **Forced Expiration.** During expiration, the patient should simulate coughing, feeling the contraction of the abdominal musculature.

These exercises can be performed while the patient is standing but it is preferable for the patient to be lying in bed to isolate the muscular area involved.

Exercises for re-activating the spine musculature in general are exercises for maintaining the position and self-extension of the back musculature, which should initially be performed on a chair and subsequently on the Swiss ball, which increases the difficulty, adding the component of proprioceptive stabilization to the merely muscular (◘ Fig. 7.2)

Both exercises can be performed with or without corset or lumbar band.

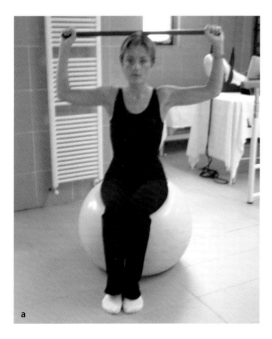 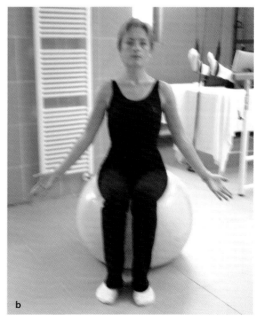

◘ **Fig. 7.2. a** THE CHANDELIER: maintenance of the position. **b** THE CROSS: maintenance of the position and self-extension

7.2 Second Stage

The second stage of the rehabilitation program starts, as already mentioned, with the stabilization of the patient and the complete healing of the wound (generally approximately 15 days after surgery), i.e. when the patient can start hydrokinesitherapy.

It is preferable to perform at least 1 hour of hydrokinesitherapy per day for 2 weeks.

The session starts with approximately 10 minutes of exercises of general warming up of the neck, upper extremities and trunk, performed in a group in the centre of the swimming pool, with the shoulders immersed in water.

It is useful to perform exercises for the articular flexibility of the cervical tract such as:
- Flexion: slowly flex the head forward expirating during flexion
- Side inclination: bring the head to the point of maximum inclination, pausing briefly in that position.
- Rotation: turn the head clockwise and then counterclockwise, up to the height of the clavicle

This is followed by exercises for the upper limbs, such as:
- Elevation: with open arms and extended elbows, raise the palms above the head; with extended elbows and interlocked fingers, raise the hands above the head.
- Opening: hands behind the nape, open and close the elbows; with open arms and extended elbows, close the arms in front of the face until the palms can be reached, and re-open.
- Rotations: with extended elbows, describe circles, first small and then increasingly large, with open arms, rotating the elbows in front and behind.

This is followed by mobilization of the spine with exercises for articular excursion and flexibility, such as:
- Bilateral flexion of the trunk
- Balancing of the pelvis
- Antero-retroversion of the pelvis

The series of exercises in the swimming pool can also include passive mobilization techniques, stretching and articular release such as those performed out of the water.

There should be also active mobilization exercises such as
- Exercises at the handrail sitting on the bench. (◘ Fig. 7.3)
- Exercises at the wall (◘ Fig. 7.4)
- Exercises in deep water (◘ Fig. 7.5a,b)

The exercises can become progressively more intense and specific for stabilization and strengthening of the lumbar musculature. Examples (◘ Fig. 7.6)

For those patients who cannot attend rehabilitation sessions in the swimming pool, the work at the gym can be supplemented using the therapy master so that active-assisted exercises and in non-weight-bearing conditions can be performed.

It is advisable that the session at the gym starts with the exercises learned during the first stage of the rehabilitation program, such as respiration with the diaphragm, and then continues with the more demanding exercises.

Some of the useful exercises at this stage are given below (◘ Fig. 7.7–7.10).

7.3 Third Stage

The third stage of the rehabilitation program, which starts after 30 days from surgery and lasts for a lifetime, consists of the patient's progressive and total return into his environment, at home, at work or just everyday social setting. The patients should become aware of how their spine works, and be given instructions on how to avoid an improper use of the spine; at the same time it is advisable for the patient to partially and progressively remove the fabric and steel corset as his physical and rehabilitative activity improves.

The relationship with the physical therapist must continue, even at longer intervals, so as to educate the patient on the self-management of his or her problem, and to lern how to avoid risks during daily efforts.

The therapist should make sure that the ergonomic instructions on sitting position and preservation of the spine are thoroughly understood and applied by the patient, while encouraging the patient to permanently return to work (with simulations, repetitions and verifications) and return to full satisfactory relationships, and helping the patient to maintain a suitable motor activity, consistent with his or her preferences.

Optional activities for maintaining a healthy spine include swimming, even at the maintenance stage, but also soft gymnastics, ball, Tai-Chi etc. can be practiced.

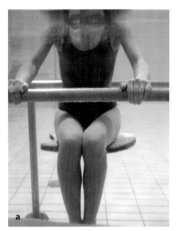
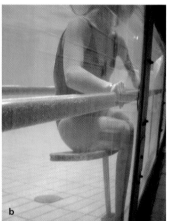
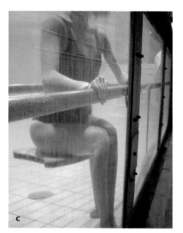
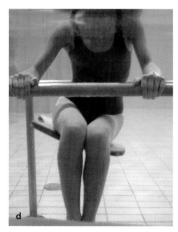
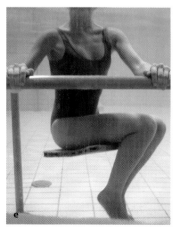

◘ **Fig. 7.3a-e.** Exercises at the handrail sitting on the bench. **a** Stabilization of the position (feet on the floor). **b,c** Antero-retroversion of the pelvis (feet on the floor). **d** Movements of lateralization of the pelvis. **e** Rotation to the right and left (with joined knees and raised feet)

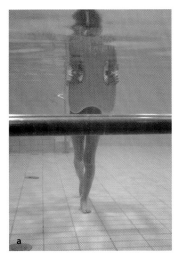
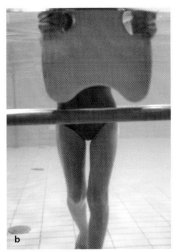
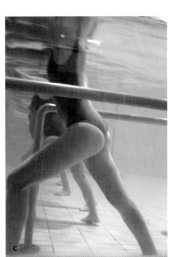

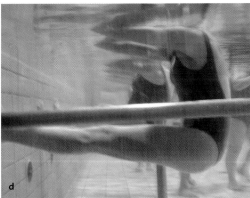

⬛ **Fig. 7.4a–d** Exercises at the wall **a** Spine on the wall: bring the knees to the chest in alternance and alternate extensions of the knees. **b** Walking forward and backwards with small steps, with or without using the bench to create attrition. **c** Hands at the edge of the swimming pool: extensions of the sural triceps. **d** Hands at the edge of the swimming pool: extensions of the flexors with feet on the wall. Hands at the edge of the swimming pool: flexion-extensions of the flexors with feet on the wall

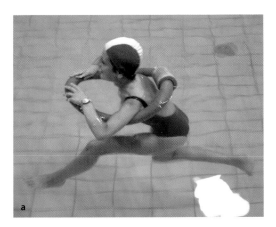
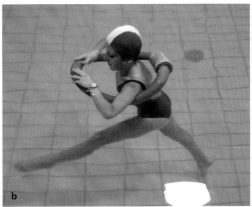

⬛ **Fig. 7.5a,b.** Exercises in deep water. In non-weight-bearing conditions with flotation device: **a** Pedalling. **b** Square opening of lower limbs

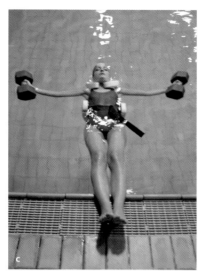
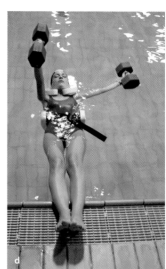

Fig. 7.5c–j. Exercises at the edge of the swimming pool. **c,d** Supine, with lumbar collar and belt, keeping the heels on the edge: opening and closing the arms with the handlebars in alternance. **e,f** Supine, with lumbar collar and belt, keeping the heels on the edge: opening and closing both arms with the handlebars. **g,h** Supine, with the thighs against the wall: strengthening of abdominal muscles. **i,j** Flat on the stomach, hands on the edge, with lumbar band and handlebar between the ankles: strengthening of lumbar muscles

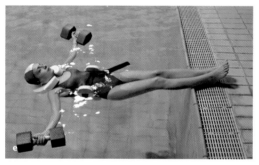
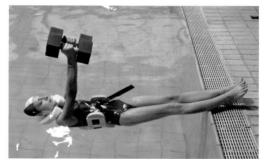
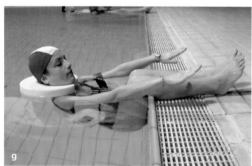
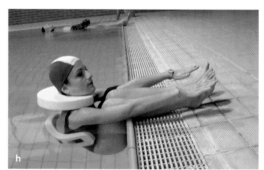
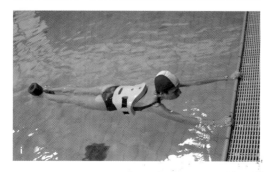
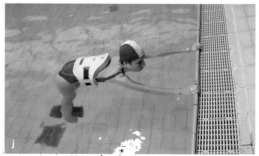

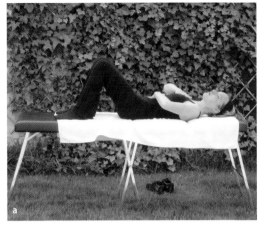

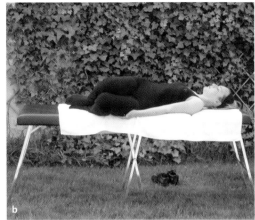

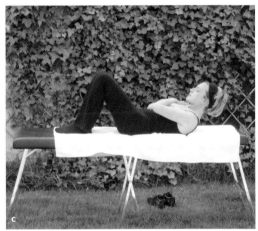

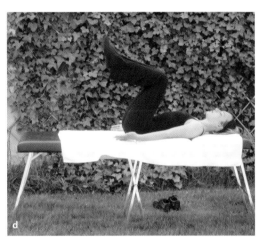

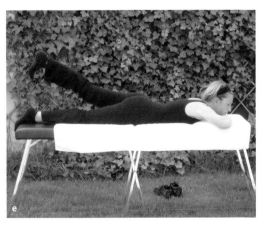

7

☐ **Fig. 7.6a–e.** Exercises on the small bed. Supine position: respiration with the diaphragm and forced expiration. **a** Supine position: inclination of the pelvis with bent knees, with the feet solidly set on the floor and arms extended along the body. At this stage, try to flatten the spine rotating the pelvis upwards. Once this position is reached, it should be maintained for a few seconds. **b** Supine position: balancing the knees from one side to the other. **c** Supine position, with bent knees, feet solidly set on the floor, and arms crossed on the chest. Keeping the lumbar and dorsal tract solidly set on the floor, raise the head and shoulders, and maintain this position for a few seconds. **d** Supine position with bent knees and feet solidly set on the floor, and arms extended along the body. At this stage, raise the knees one at a time, bring them to the chest and keep them in this position with the hands for a second. Subsequently return to original position, bringing the legs back to the floor one at a time. **e** Prone position with the arms folded under the chin and the pelvis solidly set on the small bed. Slowly raise one leg at a time, keeping it raised for a second and then slowly bring it down

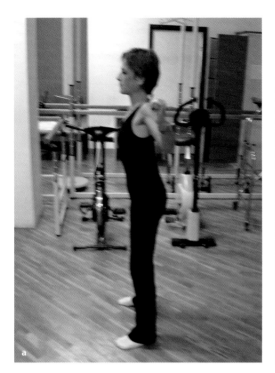

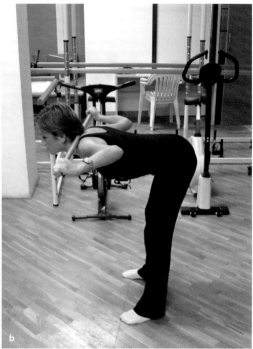

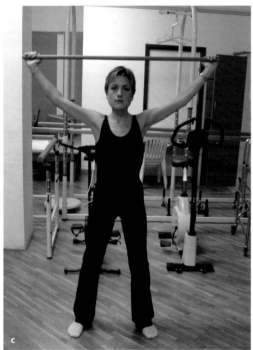

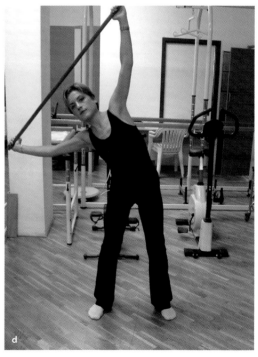

Fig. 7.7a–d. Exercises with the bar **a,b** Anterior flexion of the trunk keeping the back straight. **c,d** Lateral flexion of the trunk, keeping the bar, with extended arms, above the head

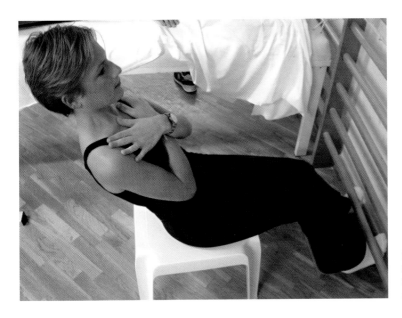

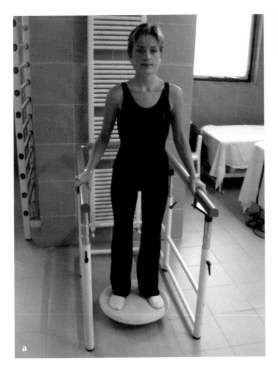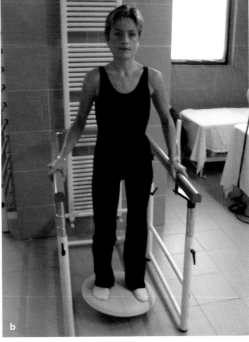

■ **Fig. 7.8.** Exercises at the espalier wall. Patient is sitting: inclination of the trunk with maintained position

a   b

■ **Fig. 7.9a,b.** Proprioceptive exercises. **a,b** On oscillating table: shifting the body weight from one leg to the other.

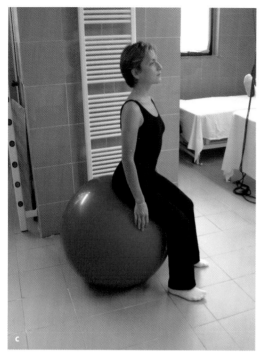

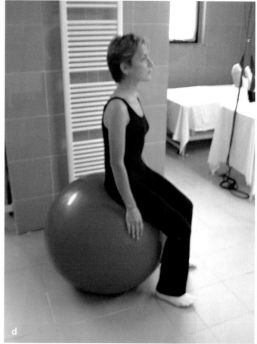

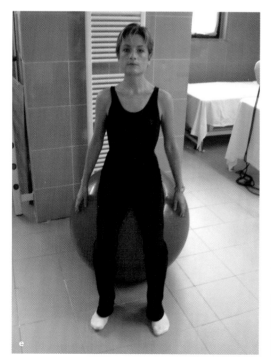

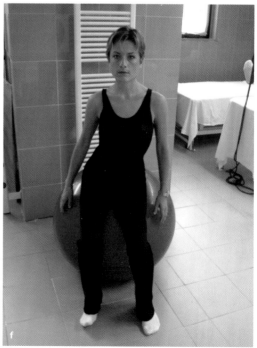

◨ **Fig. 7.9. c,d** On a ball: antero-retroversion of the pelvis. **e,f** On a ball: lateralization of the pelvis to the right and to the left.

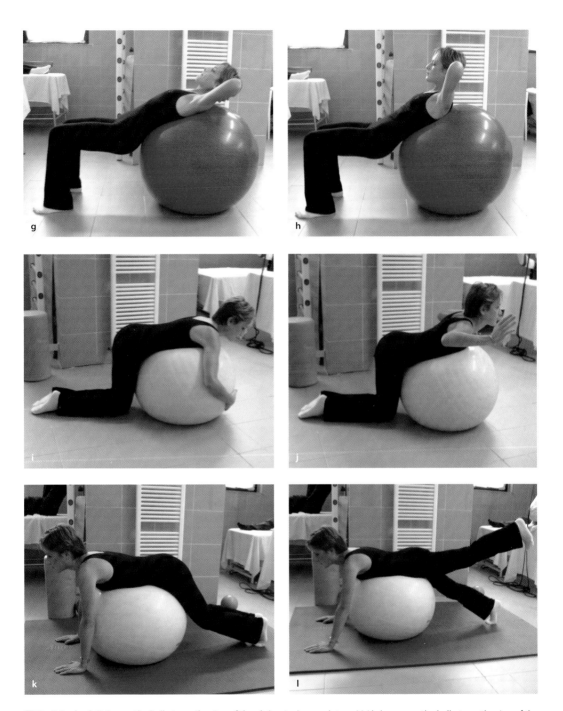

⬛ Fig. 7.9g–l. g,h Spine on the ball: strengthening of the abdominal musculature. **i,j** Abdomen on the ball: strengthening of the back musculature. **k,l** Abdomen on the ball: alternated extension of arms and legs.

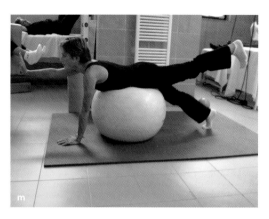

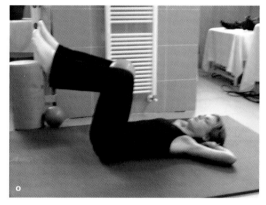

❏ **Fig. 7.9. m** Abdomen on the ball: stabilization and maintenance of the position. **n,o** Ball between the knees: bilateral
raising of the knees. **p,q** Ball between the knees: balancing the
knees from one side to the other

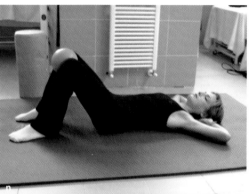

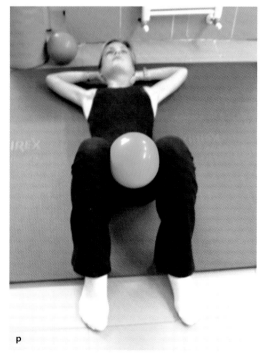

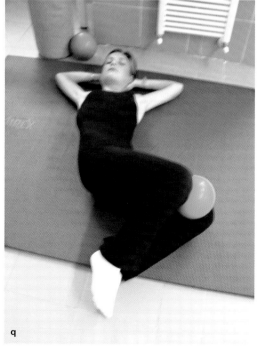

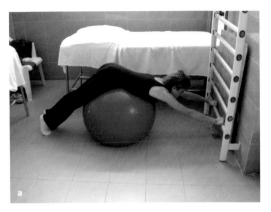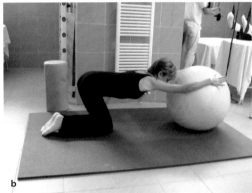

□ Fig. 7.10a,b. Stretching exercises Sitting position: static lengthening of the leg's flexor muscles
- Supine position: bring the knee to the chest and stretch using the arms
- On one's feet: lateral flexions of the trunk, accompanies by movement of the arms

a Stretching, non-weight-bearing for the spine, on Swiss ball. **b** Hands on the ball, slowly lower the pelvis towards the feet and keep the position for a second or so.

8

Conclusion

This publication is based on a review of 30 patients treated with dynamic stabilization of the lumbosacral spine with the Dynesys system, for some of them, using the Wiltse lateral approach without detachment of the muscles of the paravertebral site.

During follow-up visits, patients who underwent this surgery, assessed with the VAS evaluation scales and the Oswestry Low Back Pain Disability Questionnaire, with follow-up of 1 to 4 years, showed a significantly better and faster recovery of functionality compared with patients who had stabilization-arthrodesis. In this way, patients who, after surgery, led a physically active life, reported only a minor limitation (or none) in daily life activities in comparison with those who led a sedentary life.

With the data obtained, we can develop guidelines for the performance of a rehabilitation program specific to this surgery, by which one can accelerate recovery times and enhance the characteristics of surgery such as minimum invasiveness, restoration of the physiological functionality of the spine, and, in those cases without detachment of the paravertebral muscles (Wiltse lateral approach), return to standing position on the first day following surgery, with full restoration of the spine its function 30 days after surgery.

Acknowledgement Dr. Michele James Ceglia supervised the translation.

9

References

1. Aota Y, Kumano K, Hirabayashi S.: Postfusion instability at the adjacent segments after rigid pedicle screw fixation for degenerative lumbar spinal disorders. J Spinal Disord 1995 Dec;8(6):464-73

2. Skinner A.T., ThomsonA.M.: Tecniche Duffield, La rieducazione in acqua. Marrapese Editore, 1985

3. Cauchoix J, David T.: Lumbar arthrodesis: results after more than 10 years. Rev Chir Orthop Reparatrice Appar Mot. 1985;71(4):263-8 in French

4. Charnley J.: Physical changes in the prolapsed disc. Lancet; 1: 1277, 1958

5. Cotrell Y, Dubousset J et al.: New universal instrumentation in spinal surgery. Clin Orthop; 227, 10-23, 1998

6. Eyring EJ: Biochemistry and physiology of the intervertebral disc. Clin Orthop;67: 16, 1969

7. Dubois G: Dynamic Neutralization. A new concept for stabilization of the spine. In: Spalski M, Gunburg R, Poe MH (eds.) Lumbar segmental instability. Lippincott & Wilkins, Philadelphia 1999, pp. 233-240

8. Gillet P: The fate of the adjacent motion segments after lumbar fusion. J Spinal Disord Tech, 2003 Aug;16(4): 338-45

9. Hambly MF, Wiltse LL, Raghavan N, Schneiderman G, Koenig C.: The transition zone above a lumbosacral fusion. Spine, 1998 Aug 15;23(16):1785-92

10. Harrington PR: Treatment of scoliosis: correction and internal fixation by spine instrumentation June 1962. J Bone Joint Surg Am 2002 Feb;84-A(2):316

11. Hibbs RH: An operation for progressive spinal deformities. NY Medic J 1911,93 ; 1013

12. Kapandji IA: The functional anatomy of the lumbosacral spine. Acta Orthop Belg 1969 May-Aug;35(3):543-66

13. Kirkaldy-Willis, Wedge JH, Yong-Hing K, Tchang S, de Korompay V, Shannon R.: Lumbar spinal nerve lateral entrapment. Clin Orthop Relat Res 1982 Sep;(169):171-8

14. Kramer J, Kolditz D, Godwin R: Water and electrolyte content of human intervertebral discs under variable load. Spine 1985 Jan-Feb;10(1):69-71

15. Luque ER: Segmental spinal instrumentation of the lumbar spine. Clin Orthop Relat Res 1986 Feb(203):126-34

16. Mulholland RC, Sengupta DK: Rationale, principles and experimental evaluation of the concept of soft stabilization. Eur Spine J 2002 Oct;11 Suppl 2:S198-205. Epub 2002 Jun 4. Review

17. Macnab I: The traction spur. J Bone Joint Surg; 53: 663-670, 1971

18. Maigne R: Douleurs d'origine vertébrale et traitements par manipulations. L'expansion Scientifique, Paris 1972

19. Nachelson A, Morris J.M.: In vivo measurements of intradiscal pressure. discometry, a method for the determination of pressure in the lower lumbar discs. J Bone Joint Surg Am 1964 Jul;46:1077-92

20. Niosi CA, Zhu QA, Wilson DC, Keynan O, Wilson DR, Oxland TR: Biomechanical characterization of the three-dimensional kinematic behaviour of the Dynesys dynamic stabilization system: an in vitro study. Eur Spine J 2006 Jun;15(6):913-22. Epub 2005 Oct 11

21. Panjabi MM: Clinical spinal instability and low back pain. J Electromyography 13 (2003) 371-379

22. Roy C: Osteosynthèse du rachis dorsal, lombar, lombosacre par plaques métalliques vissées dans les pédicules vertébraux et les apophises articulaires. Presse Med 1978: 1447.1970

23. Senegas J: Mechanical supplementation by non-rigid fixation in degenerative interventetebral lumbar segment: the Wallis system. Eur Spine J 2002 OCT; 11 Suppl 2:S164-9

24. Sengupta, Dilip K, Mulholland, RC: Fulcrum assisted soft stabilization system: a new concept in the surgical treatment of degenerative low back pain. Spine 30(9):1019-1029, May 1, 2005

25. Stoll TM, Dubois G, Schwarzenbach O.: The dynamic neu-
    tralization system for the spine: a multi-center study of a
    novel non-fusion system. Eur Spine J 2002 Oct;11 Suppl 2:
    S170-8. Epub 2002 Sep 10
26. Watkins MB: Posterolateral fusion of the lumbar and
    lumbosacral spine. J Bone Joint Surg Am 1953 Oct, 35-
    A(4):1014-8
27. White AA, Panjabi MM (Eds.): Clinical biomechanics of the
    spine, 2nd ed, JB Lippincott, Philadelphia, PA, 1990
28. Wiltse LL; Bateman G; Hutchinson RH; Nelson WE: The
    paraspinal sacrospinalis-splitting approach to the lumbar
    spine. J Bone Joint Surg 50-A, NO.5, July 1968